# THE GASTRITIS HEALING RECIPES

### 50 Delicious, Gastritis-Friendly Recipes to Soothe and Heal Your Stomach

## L. G. CAPELLAN

NOTICE AND DISCLAIMER

This book and the recipes, ideas, and suggestions within are not intended as a substitute for the advice and care of your doctor. As with all new diet and nutrition regimens, the recipes in this book should be followed only after first consulting with your doctor to ensure that they are appropriate for your individual circumstances. The author is not responsible for the reader's specific health or allergy needs that may require medical supervision or for any adverse reactions to the recipes or products contained in this book. It is the reader's responsibility to ensure his or her own health and medical needs are met.

ISBN: 9798418473806

# CONTENTS

## 5 Smoothies & Beverages

# INTRODUCTION

Eating the same bland and tasteless meals every day is one of the most boring and depressing things gastritis sufferers can go through. And since it can be tricky and challenging to find gastritis-friendly recipes or to learn to cook meals that don't irritate the stomach, many of them have no choice but to stick to a boring diet.

I know how that feels and how sad it can be that, due to health concerns, you feel forced to stick to a diet that don't satisfy your taste buds, especially when you are used to eating tasty meals. It makes you feel miserable.

For me it was a pain in the butt to have to get used to eating the same tasteless chicken and mushy vegetables every day. But since I didn't know what to eat and was afraid of trying new foods, I had to stick to that boring diet for a long time.

However, eating the same foods every day eventually led me to develop nutritional deficiencies due to the lack of variety. And since I wasn't giving my body the nutrients it needed, that made my healing process much more difficult.

That is why I decided to create this book, which complements my other book, *The Gastritis Healing Book* (if you haven't read it yet you can get a FREE copy at www.lgcapellan.com/freecopy). The idea behind this book is to give you a greater variety of recipes so that you can more easily follow the gastritis diet without getting bored.

In this book, you will find 50 gluten-free and dairy-free recipes for breakfast, lunch, dinner, and snacks, which have been carefully developed to ensure that they are gastritis-friendly. To develop them, the following criteria were taken into account:

Low acid (pH higher than 5)

Low fat (less than 10g per serving)

Low salt and sugar-free

No irritating ingredients

With that said, and before we move on to the recipes, I would like to clarify a few things.

The first is that the poultry and seafood recipes, which you will find in Chapter 2, are not accompanied by any side dish. If you want to accompany one of those recipes with a side dish, you can choose any of those in Chapter 3.

However, if you choose a side dish that is not in this book, make sure it is gastritis-friendly so that you avoid irritating your stomach lining. Also, do not overdo it with the portions of the side dish, as mixing a lot of carbohydrates with proteins can delay digestion. As a general rule, the amount of carbohydrates you add to a protein-rich meal should not exceed one cup.

The second thing you should know is that in this book you will find recipes for 2 to 4 or more servings. Therefore, you must bear in mind that when preparing a recipe, you may be able to eat only 1 serving; the rest will have to be stored in the refrigerator or shared with another person. It is not advisable to eat more than one serving of those recipes that contain close to 10 grams of fat by each serving; this will help to avoid delaying digestion due to ingesting too much fat.

If you experience an increase in symptoms after you try a recipe, you may not be tolerating some new foods. The most common intolerances are to eggs, oats, bananas, and the cruciferous vegetable family—including broccoli, cauliflower, cabbage, brussels sprouts, and several others. If you suspect that you are not tolerating a particular food, remove it for a week or two and then reintroduce it.

In most cases, intolerances are related to intestinal problems, the severity of your gastritis, and a lack of gastroprotection. If this happens to you, try to protect your stomach lining as much as possible (following the suggestions in *The Gastritis Healing Book*) and increase gastroprotection naturally by consuming foods rich in linoleic acid. The latter helps to increase the production of gastric mucus. Also, do not forget to consult your doctor to rule out any other problems that may be causing food intolerances.

I really hope you like and enjoy the recipes in this book. I created them with a lot of love for you!

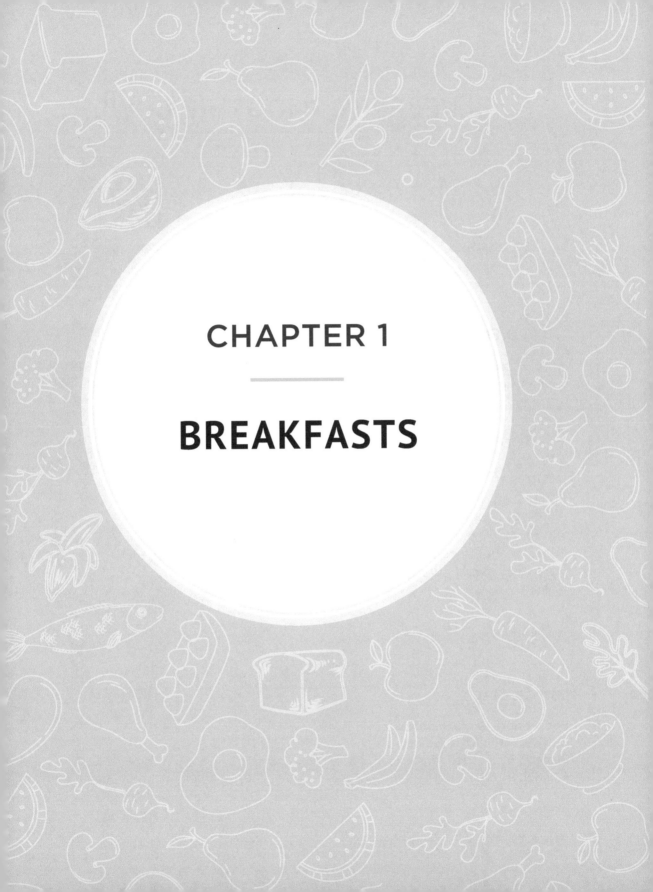

# CHAPTER 1

---

# BREAKFASTS

# BLUEBERRY SMOOTHIE BOWL

**SERVINGS**

1

**PREP TIME**

5 MIN

**COOK TIME**

N/A

## INGREDIENTS

- ⅓ - ½ cup frozen blueberries
- 2 frozen bananas, sliced
- 1 cup almond milk
- ½ tablespoon almond butter
- 1 teaspoon vanilla extract (optional)
- Toppings: coconut flakes, chia, sliced banana, maple syrup to taste

## DIRECTIONS

1. In a blender, add the almond milk, banana, blueberries, almond butter and vanilla. Blend until very smooth.

2. Pour the smoothie into a bowl.

3. Top with sliced banana or Bosc pear, coconut flakes, chia seeds and a drizzle of maple syrup, if desired.

### NUTRITION FACTS

**Per serving:** (2 cups approx.)
Calories: 365; Total fat: 8g;
Protein: 5g; Carbohydrates:
62g; Fiber: 10g

# OVERNIGHT OATS

**SERVINGS**

1

**PREP TIME**

5 MIN

**COOK TIME**

N/A

## INGREDIENTS

- ½ cup quick-cooking or unflavored instant oats
- ½ cup almond milk or other plant-based milk
- 1 teaspoon chia seeds
- 1 tablespoon maple syrup
- Toppings: ½ sliced banana and 1 tablespoon chopped walnuts.

## DIRECTIONS

1. In a small jar, combine the oats, almond milk, chia, and maple syrup.

2. Cover the glass container with a lid or plastic wrap. Let refrigerate for at least 4 hours or overnight. Toppings can be added the night before or immediately before serving.

3. Uncover and thin with a little more milk, if desired. Enjoy!

**NUTRITION FACTS**

**Per serving:** (1 cup approx.)
Calories: 339; Total fat: 9g;
Protein: 8g; Carbohydrates:
50g; Fiber: 7g

# OAT FLOUR WAFFLES

**SERVINGS**
3

**PREP TIME**
10 MIN

**COOK TIME**
20 MIN

## INGREDIENTS

- 2 cups oat flour
- 1 cup unsweetened almond milk
- 1 large egg
- 2 large egg whites
- 1 tablespoon maple syrup or honey
- 2 teaspoons baking powder
- 1 teaspoon vanilla extract
- Coconut oil for greasing
- Optional toppings: maple syrup, almond butter and/or fruits with a pH higher than 5

### NUTRITION FACTS

**Per serving:** (1 waffle)
Calories: 365; Total fat: 7g; Protein: 14g; Carbohydrates: 51g; Fiber: 8g

## DIRECTIONS

1. In a blender, combine the oat flour, almond milk, eggs, baking powder, maple syrup, and vanilla. Blend until smooth and then let the batter rest and thicken for about 10 minutes.

2. Preheat the waffle iron and grease each side with ½ teaspoon of the coconut oil or non-stick cooking spray.

3. Pour about ¾ cup of the batter onto the heated waffle iron and close the lid. Cook for 6 to 8 minutes, or until the waffle is golden brown. Remove and place waffle onto a plate or the rack of the oven (at 200°C) to keep warm.

4. Repeat with the remaining batter, greasing both sides of the waffle iron each time with the coconut oil or non-stick cooking spray.

5. Serve immediately and enjoy with your favorite toppings!

6. Store the rest of the waffles between parchment paper in the fridge for up to 4 days or in the freezer for up to 2 months. For best results, reheat waffles in the toaster oven.

# PUMPKIN PANCAKES

**SERVINGS**
2

**PREP TIME**
5 MIN

**COOK TIME**
10 MIN

## INGREDIENTS

- 1 large egg, beaten
- 1 egg white
- ½ cup pumpkin puree (not pumpkin pie filling)
- ½ cup gluten free all-purpose flour (see note)
- ½ teaspoon grated fresh ginger (optional)

## DIRECTIONS

1. In a medium bowl, whisk together the eggs, pumpkin, flour, and ginger.
2. Grease a large nonstick skillet with coconut oil or non-stick cooking spray and place over medium-high heat. Once the pan is hot, pour about ¼ cup of the batter onto the skillet.
3. Cook until bubbles form on the top or until the bottom is golden-brown, about 2 to 3 minutes. Flip and cook 3 minutes more on the other side.

## NUTRITION FACTS

**Per serving:** (2 pancakes) Calories: 243; Total fat: 4g; Protein: 7g; Carbohydrates: 34g; Fiber: 11g

## NOTE

You can substitute the gluten free all-purpose flour with gluten free pancake mix or oat flour.

# BANANA AVOCADO SMOOTHIE

**SERVINGS**

1

**PREP TIME**

5 MIN

**COOK TIME**

N/A

## INGREDIENTS

- 1 ripe banana
- ¼ cup avocado, peeled and pitted
- 1 ½ cups almond milk
- 1 tablespoon maple syrup
- ½ teaspoon fresh ginger, grated (optional)

## DIRECTIONS

1. Place all the ingredients in a blender and blend until smooth.
2. Serve immediately and enjoy!

**NUTRITION FACTS**

**Per serving:** (2 cups) Calories: 280; Total fat: 9.6g; Protein: 4g; Carbohydrates: 42g; Fiber: 7g

# GLUTEN-FREE FRENCH TOAST

**SERVINGS**
2

**PREP TIME**
10 MIN

**COOK TIME**
10 MIN

## INGREDIENTS

- 1 large egg, beaten
- 1 egg white
- ½ cup almond milk
- ½ teaspoon vanilla extract
- 4 slices gluten-free bread
- Pinch of salt
- ¼ teaspoon cinnamon powder (optional, if tolerated)

## DIRECTIONS

1. In a medium bowl, whisk together the eggs, almond milk, vanilla, salt, and cinnamon (if tolerated).

2. Pour the mixture into a shallow dish. Soak the bread in the mixture until the liquid is absorbed, about 3 minutes per side.

3. Grease a large nonstick skillet with coconut oil or non-stick cooking spray and place over medium-high heat. Once hot, add the bread and cook until the custard sets, about 3 to 4 minutes per side.

4. Serve warm with maple syrup (or other toppings of your choice) and enjoy!

**NUTRITION FACTS**

**Per serving:** (2 slices)
Calories: 205; Total fat: 7g;
Protein: 6.5g; Carbohydrates:
27g; Fiber: 1g

# TURKEY BREAKFAST SAUSAGE

**SERVINGS**
2

**PREP TIME**
10 MIN

**COOK TIME**
15 MIN

## INGREDIENTS

- 8 ounces ground turkey
- 2 teaspoons ground sage
- ½ teaspoon dried thyme
- ½ teaspoon sea salt
- 1 tablespoon olive oil

## DIRECTIONS

1. In a medium bowl, combine the ground turkey, sage, thyme, and salt. Mix well.
2. Form the mixture into about 4 patties.
3. Grease a large nonstick skillet with the olive oil and place over medium-high heat. Once the oil shimmers, add the patties and cook until browned on both sides, about 4 minutes per side.
4. Place patties on a paper towel-lined plate to drain any excess oil. Serve and enjoy!

**NUTRITION FACTS**

**Per serving:** (1 patty)
Calories: 120; Total fat: 6.5g;
Protein: 15g; Carbohydrates:
0g; Fiber: 0g

**NOTE**

You can make a double the batch and freeze. Wrap each patty in plastic wrap and then place in a zip lock bag or resealable freezer bag. They'll keep for up to 3 months in the freezer.

# PUMPKIN HARVEST HASH

**SERVINGS**

2

**PREP TIME**

25 MIN

**COOK TIME**

25 MIN

## INGREDIENTS

- ½ pound ground turkey
- ½ cup pumpkin, cubed
- 1 cup kale, chopped
- 1 cup mushrooms, diced
- 2 tablespoons chicken or vegetable broth (optional)
- ½ teaspoon dried oregano
- ½ teaspoon asafoetida (optional)
- 1 tablespoon olive oil
- ½ teaspoon salt
- 1 sprig fresh thyme
- 2 teaspoons fresh chopped sage

### NUTRITION FACTS

**Per serving:** (1 small bowl approx.) Calories: 162; Total fat: 9g; Protein: 17g; Carbohydrates: 3g; Fiber: 2g

## DIRECTIONS

1. In a small bowl, combine the salt, oregano and asafoetida (optional).

2. Heat a medium skillet over medium heat and add the turkey and the seasoning mixture to the skillet. Cook until browned, stirring occasionally and breaking into crumbles. Set aside.

3. Grease the same skillet with the olive oil and then add the diced mushrooms and fresh thyme leaves. Cook for about 2 minutes, stirring occasionally. Add the cubed pumpkin and seasoning with salt. Cook, stirring occasionally, until the pumpkin is tender.

4. Once the pumpkin is tender, add the ground turkey that you set aside back to the skillet. Add 2 tablespoons of chicken or vegetable broth (optional) and the fresh sage to the skillet and reduce heat to a simmer. Cook for about 2 to 3 more minutes. Stir in chopped kale and cook until wilted.

5. Serve and enjoy!

# BLUEBERRY CHIA PUDDING

**SERVINGS**

1

**PREP TIME**

10 MIN

**COOK TIME**

N/A

## INGREDIENTS

- ½ cup almond milk
- 2 tablespoons chia seeds
- ¼ cup fresh blueberries
- 1 tablespoon maple syrup
- ½ teaspoon vanilla extract (optional)

## DIRECTIONS

1. Place the almond milk and blueberries in a blender and blend until smooth.

2. Pour the mixture into sealable jar or a bowl. Add in the chia seeds, maple syrup, and vanilla. Mix well.

3. Let sit for about 10 minutes, then mix the pudding again to break up any clumping.

4. Place in the fridge for a minimum of 2 hours, or preferably overnight. Stir the mixture again before serving and top as desired. Enjoy!

**NUTRITION FACTS**

**Per serving:** (1 cup) Calories: 198; Total fat: 7.5g; Protein: 4g; Carbohydrates: 23g; Fiber: 8g

# CREAM OF RICE CEREAL

**SERVINGS**
1

**PREP TIME**
10 MIN

**COOK TIME**
15 MIN

## INGREDIENTS

- ½ cup uncooked white rice
- 2 ¼ cups almond milk
- Pinch of salt
- Optional toppings: banana slices, coconut flakes, or chopped walnuts and/or maple syrup.

## DIRECTIONS

1. In a blender or coffee grinder, grind the rice coarsely.
2. In a medium saucepan, add the almond milk and bring to a low boil, stirring constantly to prevent burning.
3. Stir in the rice and salt.
4. Cover and simmer for about 5 to 15 minutes, until thickened. Watch the pan when cooking the rice. Add more liquid if needed to keep it from sticking to the bottom of the pan.
5. Serve with toppings.

**NUTRITION FACTS**

**Per serving:** (2 cups approx.)
Calories: 468; Total fat: 6g; Protein: 8g; Carbohydrates: 89g; Fiber: 4g

# CHAPTER 2

## POULTRY AND SEAFOOD

# SWEET POTATO CHICKEN NUGGETS

**SERVINGS**
2

**PREP TIME**
15 MIN

**COOK TIME**
10 MIN

## INGREDIENTS

- ½ pound ground chicken breast
- 1 cup sweet potato, shredded (see note)
- 1 tablespoon coconut flour
- 2 teaspoons coconut oil
- ½ teaspoon salt

## DIRECTIONS

1. Preheat the oven to 400 degrees F. and grease a baking sheet with a little bit of coconut oil or non-stick cooking spray.

2. In a large mixing bowl, add the ground chicken, shredded sweet potato, coconut oil, and coconut flour and thoroughly combine.

3. Using your hands, roll the mixture into small, slightly flattened nugget shapes about 1-inch in diameter. Place each formed nugget directly onto the greased baking sheet.

4. Place in the oven for about 8 to 10 minutes, or until the chicken is fully cooked, flipping halfway through. Remove from the oven when thoroughly cooked through.

5. Serve warm and enjoy!

**NOTE**

You can use a food processor to shred the sweet potato.

**NUTRITION FACTS**

**Per serving:** (about 6 nuggets) Calories: 283; Total fat: 8g; Protein: 28g; Carbohydrates: 23g; Fiber: 4g

# HERB SHRIMP PASTA

**SERVINGS**
4

**PREP TIME**
15 MIN

**COOK TIME**
20 MIN

## INGREDIENTS

- 1 pound shrimp, peeled and deveined
- 8 ounces gluten-free pasta (preferably angel hair pasta)
- 2 teaspoons dried basil
- 1 teaspoon dried oregano
- 1 tablespoon olive oil
- ½ teaspoon salt
- ¼ cup grated dairy-free parmesan cheese

## DIRECTIONS

1. Boil water in a medium saucepan and cook the pasta according to package directions.

2. Grease a large skillet with a little bit of olive oil or non-stick cooking spray. Place over medium-high heat, and add the tablespoon of olive oil.

3. Add the oregano, basil, salt, and shrimp. Toss to coat shrimp with herbs and cook for about 6 to 8 minutes, or until shrimp are cooked and turn pink, turning once.

4. Drain the pasta and toss shrimp mixture with hot pasta. Sprinkle with the dairy-free parmesan cheese and serve.

### NUTRITION FACTS

**Per serving:** (1 ½ cups each)
Calories: 374; Total fat: 5g;
Protein: 29g; Carbohydrates:
45g; Fiber: 2g

# ALMOND CRUSTED CHICKEN

**SERVINGS**

2

**PREP TIME**

15 MIN

**COOK TIME**

20 MIN

## INGREDIENTS

- 1 egg, beaten
- 1 boneless, skinless chicken breast
- ½ cup blanched almond flour
- ½ teaspoon dried oregano
- ¼ teaspoon dried basil
- ½ teaspoon salt
- Olive oil for drizzling

## DIRECTIONS

1. Preheat the oven to 375 degrees F. and line a baking sheet with parchment paper.
2. In a small bowl, mix together the oregano, basil, salt, and almond flour and then spread the mixture onto a plate or a shallow bowl.
3. Pour the beaten egg in a shallow bowl.
4. Dredge the chicken in the egg and then in the almond flour mixture, coating both sides.
5. Place the chicken on the lined baking sheet with parchment paper. Drizzle a little bit of oil over top of chicken to help make crispy.
6. Bake for about 10-15 minutes on one side, flip and bake for another 10 minutes, or until golden brown. Serve warm.

**NUTRITION FACTS**

**Per serving:** (½ chicken breast) Calories: 198; Total fat: 9g; Protein: 24g; Carbohydrates: 1g; Fiber: 1g

**NOTE**

If desired, you can cut the chicken breast into ½-inch thick strips lengthwise.

# SIMPLE SALMON CAKES

**SERVINGS**

4

**PREP TIME**

15 MIN

**COOK TIME**

10 MIN

## INGREDIENTS

- 1 can (14.75 oz) salmon, drained
- ⅔ cup gluten-free breadcrumbs
- 1 egg, beaten
- 1 teaspoon dried dill
- ½ teaspoon lemon zest, grated (optional)
- ½ teaspoon asafoetida (optional, but recommended)
- ½ teaspoon salt
- 2 teaspoons olive oil

## DIRECTIONS

1. In a medium bowl, mix all the ingredients together, except the olive oil.

2. Using your hands, form 4 evenly-sized patties.

3. In a large skillet over medium heat, heat the olive oil. Add the patties to the skillet and cook until golden brown on each side, about 3-5 minutes per side.

4. Serve the salmon patties with the side dish of your choice.

**NUTRITION FACTS**

**Per serving:** (1 patty)
Calories: 230; Total fat: 4g;
Protein: 26g; Carbohydrates:
14g; Fiber: 0g

# GROUND TURKEY STROGANOFF

**SERVINGS**
4

**PREP TIME**
10 MIN

**COOK TIME**
20 MIN

## INGREDIENTS

- 1 lb. ground turkey breast
- 8 oz. mushrooms, sliced
- 1 cup unsweetened almond milk
- 1 ¼ cups chicken broth
- 1 tablespoon Bragg liquid aminos or coconut aminos
- 2 tablespoons parsley, chopped
- 1 teaspoon dried thyme
- 1 teaspoon asafoetida (optional)
- 2 tablespoons arrowroot flour or cornstarch
- 2 teaspoons olive oil

### NUTRITION FACTS

**Per serving:** (¾ cup approx.)
Calories: 176; Total fat: 6g;
Protein: 28g; Carbohydrates:
4.7g; Fiber: 1g

## DIRECTIONS

1. Heat 1 teaspoon of olive oil in a skillet over medium heat. Place the turkey in the skillet and cook, stirring occasionally, until crumbled and browned, about 5 to 7 minutes. Remove from skillet and set aside.

2. Add to the skillet the mushrooms and 1 teaspoon of olive oil, cook for about 3-5 minutes or until mushrooms are tender.

3. While mushrooms are cooking, add the almond milk to a medium bowl and whisk in the arrowroot or cornstarch, making sure there are no lumps.

4. After mushrooms are done, add the vegetable broth, liquid aminos, thyme, asafoetida, and almond milk mixture to the skillet with the mushrooms. Simmer for about 10 minutes allowing for the sauce to thicken.

5. Add the turkey and parsley and simmer for another 5-8 minutes. Season with salt to taste.

6. Serve over cooked rice or pasta.

# SEARED SCALLOPS WITH SPINACH

**SERVINGS**

2

**PREP TIME**

5 MIN

**COOK TIME**

10 MIN

## INGREDIENTS

- 8 ounces scallops
- 1 tablespoon olive oil
- ¼ teaspoon salt
- 1 ½ cups baby spinach
- 1 teaspoon lemon zest

## DIRECTIONS

1. Heat a medium skillet over medium-high heat and grease it with the olive oil.
2. Season the scallops with salt.
3. Once the oil shimmers, carefully place the scallops one by one in the pan. Cook for about 2 minutes, then flip the scallops using tongs and cook for 1 more minute, or until browned on each side. Remove the scallops from the pan.
4. Add the spinach and orange zest to the pan and cook, stirring frequently, until the spinach wilts, about 2 to 3 minutes.
5. Serve and enjoy!

**NUTRITION FACTS**

**Per serving:** (½ of recipe)
Calories: 171; Total fat: 5.5g;
Protein: 24g; Carbohydrates:
6g; Fiber: 1g

# BROILED CHICKEN KABOBS

**SERVINGS**

2

**PREP TIME**

20 MIN

**COOK TIME**

10 MIN

## INGREDIENTS

- 2 boneless, skinless chicken breasts, cut into 1-inch pieces
- 2 cups zucchini, cut into 1-inch pieces
- 1 ½ cups whole button mushrooms, stems removed
- 2 teaspoons olive oil
- ½ teaspoon dried oregano
- ½ teaspoon dried basil
- ¼ teaspoon dried rosemary
- ¼ teaspoon fresh parsley
- ¼ teaspoon salt

### NUTRITION FACTS

**Per serving:** (⅓ of recipe)
Calories: 192; Total fat: 7g;
Protein: 27g; Carbohydrates:
2.6g; Fiber: 1g

## DIRECTIONS

1. In a medium bowl, combine the oregano, basil, rosemary, parsley, salt, and olive oil.
2. Add the chicken pieces to the bowl and toss well to coat. Let sit for 5 minutes.
3. Turn the broiler on and preheat for 15 to 20 minutes.
4. Stir button mushrooms and zucchini pieces into the bowl of the chicken mixture.
5. Thread the chicken, zucchini pieces, and mushrooms alternating them onto skewers.
6. Prepare a baking sheet by lining it with foil or spray it with non-stick cooking spray. Arrange the kabobs in a single layer.
7. Place the baking sheet under broil and broil for about 5 minutes on each side, turning once.
8. Serve with the side dish of your choice.

# CRAB CAKES

**SERVINGS**
2

**PREP TIME**
10 MIN

**COOK TIME**
15 MIN

## INGREDIENTS

- 8 ounces lump crab meat, drained
- ⅔ cup gluten-free breadcrumbs
- 1 large egg, beaten
- 2 tablespoons chopped fresh cilantro
- 1 teaspoon lime zest
- ¼ teaspoon salt

## DIRECTIONS

1. Preheat the oven to 450 degrees F. and grease a rimmed baking sheet with a little bit of olive oil or non-stick cooking spray.

2. In a medium bowl, combine the crab, egg, breadcrumbs, cilantro, lime zest, and salt. Cover and refrigerate for 25 minutes.

3. Remove crab mixture from fridge and form into two or three crab cakes. Place them on the prepared baking sheet and bake for about 15 minutes, or until golden brown.

4. Serve with the side dish of your choice.

**NUTRITION FACTS**

**Per serving:** (½ of recipe)
Calories: 261; Total fat: 3g;
Protein: 25g; Carbohydrates:
29g; Fiber: 0g

# SWEET POTATO NOODLES SKILLET

**SERVINGS**
4

**PREP TIME**
15 MIN

**COOK TIME**
15 MIN

## INGREDIENTS

- 1 pound ground turkey breast
- 1 medium sweet potato, spiralized (see note)
- 1 cup baby spinach
- 1 tablespoon olive oil
- ½ teaspoon dried oregano
- ½ teaspoon ground cumin
- Salt to taste

## DIRECTIONS

1. Heat the olive oil in a skillet over medium heat. Add the ground turkey to the skillet and season with the salt, oregano, and cumin.

2. Halfway through cooking the ground turkey, add the sweet potato noodles and cook for about 5 to 8 minutes, tossing with a spatula. You can add a few tablespoons of water to prevent noodles from sticking.

3. Add in the baby spinach and cook for about 2 more minutes, or until the spinach is wilted.

4. Serve warm and enjoy!

**NUTRITION FACTS**

**Per serving:** (¾ cup approx.)
Calories: 192; Total fat: 4g;
Protein: 26g; Carbohydrates:
4g; Fiber: 1g

**NOTE**

You can use a spiralizer to make your own sweet potato noodles or alternatively buy a package in the supermarket.

# EASY BAKED COD

**SERVINGS**

2

**PREP TIME**

5 MIN

**COOK TIME**

12 MIN

## INGREDIENTS

- 2 (4-ounce) cod fillets
- 1 tablespoon fresh dill, chopped
- ½ teaspoon grated lemon zest
- ¼ teaspoon sea salt
- 1 teaspoon olive oil

## DIRECTIONS

1. Preheat the oven to 400 degrees F. and line a rimmed baking sheet with parchment paper.

2. In a medium bowl, mix together the olive oil, dill, lemon zest, and salt. Add the cod fillets and coat with the oil mixture.

3. Place the cod on the prepared baking sheet and bake until the fish is flaky and opaque, about 10 to 12 minutes.

4. Serve with the side dish of your choice.

**NUTRITION FACTS**

**Per serving:** (1 cod fillet)
Calories: 147; Total fat: 7g;
Protein: 20g; Carbohydrates:
0g; Fiber: 0g

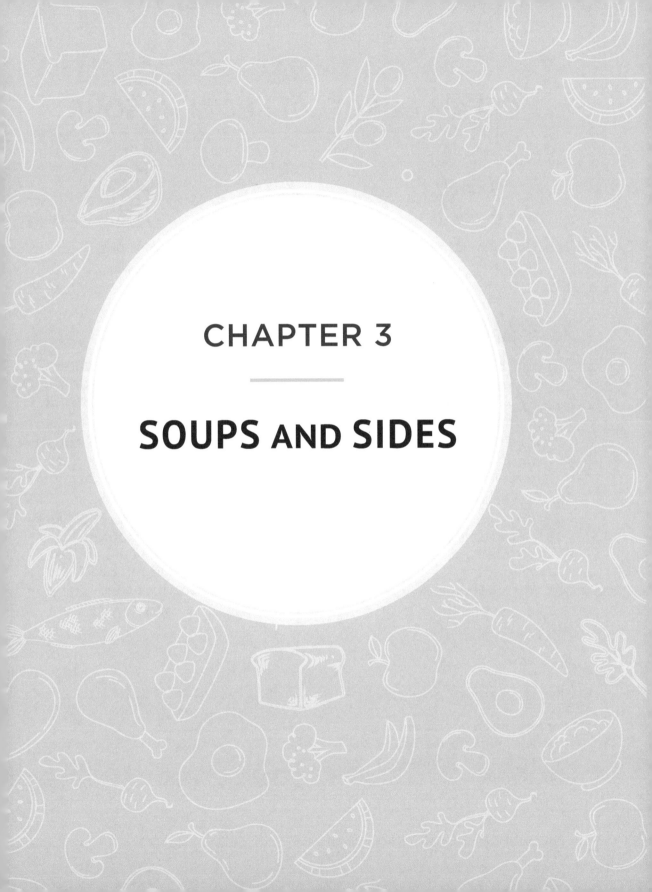

# CHAPTER 3

## SOUPS AND SIDES

# CREAMY BROCCOLI POTATO SOUP

**SERVINGS**
2

**PREP TIME**
20 MIN

**COOK TIME**
20 MIN

## INGREDIENTS

- 3 cups broccoli, chopped
- 4 medium potatoes, peeled and cubed
- 1 cup carrots, shredded
- 2 cups water or vegetable broth
- ⅓ cup canned coconut milk
- 2 tablespoons of arrowroot flour or cornstarch
- ¼ cup nutritional yeast
- ¼ teaspoon salt

## DIRECTIONS

1. In a medium stockpot, bring the water or vegetable broth to a boil and add the potatoes, broccoli, carrots, and salt. Let cook for about 15 minutes.

2. While vegetables are cooking, mix together the arrowroot, coconut milk and ¼ cup water (you can use a blender for a smooth consistency). Set aside.

3. Once the vegetables are finished cooking, let simmer and add the coconut milk mixture. Stir in nutritional yeast and let cook another minute, and remove from heat. Add salt to taste, if desired. Enjoy!

**NUTRITION FACTS**

**Per serving:** (½ of recipe)
Calories: 445; Total fat: 7g;
Protein: 17g; Carbohydrates:
63g; Fiber: 17g

# CHICKEN AND CAULIFLOWER RICE SOUP

**SERVINGS**

2

**PREP TIME**

20 MIN

**COOK TIME**

25 MIN

## INGREDIENTS

- 1 boneless, skinless chicken breast
- 3 cups riced cauliflower (see note)
- 2 medium carrots, sliced
- 2 celery stalks, sliced
- 3 cups of chicken broth
- 2 cups of water
- 1 tablespoon olive oil
- ½ teaspoon ground turmeric
- ¼ teaspoon asafetida (optional)
- 1 bay leaf
- 1 tablespoon chopped thyme leaves

## DIRECTIONS

1. Bring the broth and water to a boil in a stockpot and then add the chicken breast, carrots, celery, bay leaf, salt, asafoetida (optional), and chopped thyme leaves. Lower the heat to a simmer and cover with a lid.

2. While the vegetables and chicken are cooking, heat a skillet over medium heat and add the olive oil. When the oil is hot add the riced cauliflower, ground turmeric, and salt to taste. Cook for about 10 minutes, stirring occasionally.

3. Once the vegetables are tender and the chicken is cooked through, remove the chicken from the stockpot and shred it with a fork. Add the shredded chicken and turmeric cauliflower rice to the stockpot. Season with salt to taste and enjoy!

## NUTRITION FACTS

**Per serving:** (½ of recipe) Calories: 217; Total fat: 8g; Protein: 22g; Carbohydrates: 7g; Fiber: 7g

## NOTE

If using a box grater, cut the cauliflower into chunks and use the medium-sized holes, to grate into "rice." And if using a food processor, cut into small pieces and use the grater attachment to grate the cauliflower into "rice."

# GINGER AND TURMERIC CARROT SOUP

**SERVINGS**
2

**PREP TIME**
15 MIN

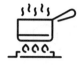

**COOK TIME**
30 MIN

## INGREDIENTS

- 3 cups carrots, chopped
- 1 leek (white part only), sliced
- 1 cup fennel, chopped
- 1 cup butternut squash, chopped
- 3 cups vegetable broth
- ½ cup lite coconut milk
- 1 tablespoon olive oil
- 1 tablespoon grated ginger
- 1 tablespoon turmeric powder
- ½ teaspoon asafoetida (optional)
- Salt to taste

### NUTRITION FACTS

**Per serving:** (½ of recipe)
Calories: 220; Total fat: 8g;
Protein: 4g; Carbohydrates:
25g; Fiber: 10g

## DIRECTIONS

1. Heat the olive oil in a large saucepan. Add the carrots, leeks, squash, and fennel. Sauté for about 3 to 5 minutes until the vegetables start to soften. Add the ginger, turmeric, and salt to taste, and sauté for a few more minutes.

2. Add the broth and coconut milk and bring the mixture to a boil, cover with the lid and simmer for about 20 minutes.

3. Once the soup is ready, add it to a blender and blend until smooth and creamy. Alternatively, you can use an immersion blender. Taste and season with salt to taste.

4. Serve immediately and enjoy!

# BUTTERNUT SQUASH SOUP

**SERVINGS**

2

**PREP TIME**

20 MIN

**COOK TIME**

35 MIN

## INGREDIENTS

- 1 butternut squash, peeled and cubed
- 2 medium carrots, chopped
- 2 celery stalks, roughly chopped
- ½ leek (white part only), washed and sliced
- 3 ½ cups vegetable broth or water
- ½ cup unsweetened coconut milk or other plant-based milk
- 2 teaspoon olive oil
- ¾ teaspoon of sage
- ½ teaspoon salt

## DIRECTIONS

1. Heat the olive oil in a large stockpot over medium-high heat. Add the leek, carrot, and celery and sauté for about 5 minutes. Lower the heat if the vegetable vegetables begin to brown.

2. Add the butternut squash, broth, salt, and sage into the stockpot and bring to a boil. Then reduce to a simmer, cover, and cook for 20 to 30 minutes, until the squash and carrots have softened. Remove and discard the sage. Stir in the coconut milk.

3. Use an immersion blender to purée the soup, or alternatively, work in batches and purée the soup in a stand blender.

4. Taste and season the soup with salt as needed. Serve warm and enjoy!

### NUTRITION FACTS

**Per serving:** (½ of recipe)
Calories: 293; Total fat: 7g;
Protein: 5.5g; Carbohydrates:
42g; Fiber: 17g

# CREAMY CHICKEN KALE SOUP

**SERVINGS**
2

**PREP TIME**
20 MIN

**COOK TIME**
30 MIN

## INGREDIENTS

- 1 boneless, skinless chicken breast
- 1-2 cups kale, roughly cut
- 1 ½ cups carrots, peeled and diced
- 1 ½ cups celery, diced
- 8 oz. baby bella mushrooms, sliced
- 5 cups chicken or vegetable broth
- 1 tablespoon fresh thyme
- 2-3 tablespoons of arrowroot flour or cornstarch
- ⅓ cup lite coconut milk
- 1 teaspoon olive oil

### NUTRITION FACTS

**Per serving:** (½ of recipe)
Calories: 243; Total fat: 8g;
Protein: 27g; Carbohydrates:
10g; Fiber: 6g

## DIRECTIONS

1. Heat the olive oil in a large dutch oven or stockpot over medium-high heat. Add the carrots and celery. Season with salt and sauté for 3 minutes. Add the fresh thyme and mushrooms and give a quick toss.

2. Add the broth and chicken to the dutch oven and bring to a boil. Lower the heat to a simmer and cover the pot with a lid and cook until the vegetables turn soft, but not mushy.

3. In a medium bowl, mix together the arrowroot flour or cornstarch, coconut milk and ¼ cup water until there are no lumps. You can use a blender for a smooth consistency. Set aside.

4. Once the vegetables are tender and the chicken is cooked through, remove the chicken from the stockpot and shred it with a fork. Add the shredded chicken to the pot and pour the arrowroot/milk mixture into the soup. Taste and add more salt if desired.

5. Add kale and stir well. Let the soup simmer a few minutes before serving. Enjoy!

# MASHED RUTABAGA

**SERVINGS**
2

**PREP TIME**
10 MIN

**COOK TIME**
35 MIN

## INGREDIENTS

- 2 medium rutabagas, peeled and chopped into 1-inch chunks
- 1 tablespoon olive oil
- ½ teaspoon salt
- 1 tablespoon chopped parsley

## DIRECTIONS

1. In a large saucepan, place the chopped rutabaga and cover with about 1 inch of water. Add the salt and boil until tender, about 25 to 35 minutes.

2. Drain the water and add the olive oil. Mash the rutabagas using a fork or potato masher.

3. Taste and add more salt if desired. Top with fresh chopped parsley.

**NUTRITION FACTS**

**Per serving:** (1 cup approx.)
Calories: 202; Total fat: 4g;
Protein: 4g; Carbohydrates:
7g; Fiber: 8g

# MUSHROOM RICE

**SERVINGS**

2

**PREP TIME**

10 MIN

**COOK TIME**

15 MIN

## INGREDIENTS

- 6 oz. mushrooms, sliced
- 1 cup uncooked white rice
- 2 cups vegetable or chicken broth
- 1 teaspoon olive oil
- 6-8 sprigs thyme
- Salt to taste

## DIRECTIONS

1. Heat the olive oil in a saucepan over medium-high heat and add the mushrooms and sauté for about 4 to 5 minutes. Season with salt and thyme leaves. Set half the mushrooms aside.

2. Add the rice to saucepan along with bone broth and bring to a boil. Once the water starts to evaporate, reduce the heat to low. Stir and cook covered for about 10-15 minutes.

3. Stir in remaining mushrooms, and season with salt and thyme to taste.

**NUTRITION FACTS**

**Per serving:** (1 cup approx.)
Calories: 376; Total fat: 3g;
Protein: 9g; Carbohydrates: 73g; Fiber: 2g

# ROASTED BROCCOLI

**SERVINGS**

2

**PREP TIME**

10 MIN

**COOK TIME**

22 MIN

## INGREDIENTS

- 6 ounces broccoli, cut into florets
- 2 teaspoons olive oil
- ¼ cup grated dairy-free parmesan cheese (optional)
- Salt to taste

## DIRECTIONS

1. Preheat the oven to 400 degrees F. and line a baking sheet with parchment paper or grease it with a little bit of oil.
2. Toss the broccoli florets with olive oil and salt, and spread evenly on the baking sheet.
3. Roast for 15 to 22 minutes or until browned around the edges. Sprinkle with dairy-free parmesan cheese (optional).

**NUTRITION FACTS**

**Per serving:** (1 cup approx.)
Calories: 96; Total fat: 6g;
Protein: 5.5g; Carbohydrates:
4g; Fiber: 2g

# SAUTÉED BRUSSELS SPROUTS

**SERVINGS**

2

**PREP TIME**

10 MIN

**COOK TIME**

10 MIN

## INGREDIENTS

- 6 ounces Brussels sprouts, shredded or julienned
- 1 tablespoon olive oil
- ½ teaspoon sea salt
- ¼ cup grated dairy-free Parmesan cheese (optional)

## DIRECTIONS

1. Heat the olive oil in a non-stick skillet over medium-high heat.
2. As soon as the oil is hot and shining, swirl to cost the pan, then add the Brussels sprouts and salt. Cook, stirring occasionally, until the sprouts are browned all over and just turning tender the inside, about 6 to 8 minutes.
3. Remove from the heat and toss with ¼ cup grated dairy-free Parmesan cheese (optional) before serving. Enjoy!

**NUTRITION FACTS**

**Per serving:** (1 cup approx.)
Calories: 124; Total fat: 8g;
Protein: 6g; Carbohydrates:
5g; Fiber: 3g

# MASHED SWEET POTATOES

**SERVINGS**

2

**PREP TIME**

10 MIN

**COOK TIME**

20 MIN

## INGREDIENTS

- 2 medium sweet potatoes, peeled and cut into 1-inch pieces
- ½ cup almond milk or other plant-based milk
- ¼ cup dairy-free plain yogurt (optional)
- 1 teaspoon grated fresh ginger
- ½ teaspoon salt

## DIRECTIONS

1. Place the sweet potatoes in a large saucepan and cover with at least 1-inch of water. Place over medium-high heat and bring to a boil.

2. Cover with a lid and cook until the sweet potatoes are tender, about 15-20 minutes.

3. Drain the water and return the sweet potatoes to the saucepan. Add the ginger, milk, yogurt (optional), and salt.

4. Mash with a potato masher until smooth, and then stir well to combine. Serve immediately.

**NUTRITION FACTS**

**Per serving:** (½ cup approx.)
Calories: 148; Total fat: 2g;
Protein: 2g; Carbohydrates:
28g; Fiber: 4g

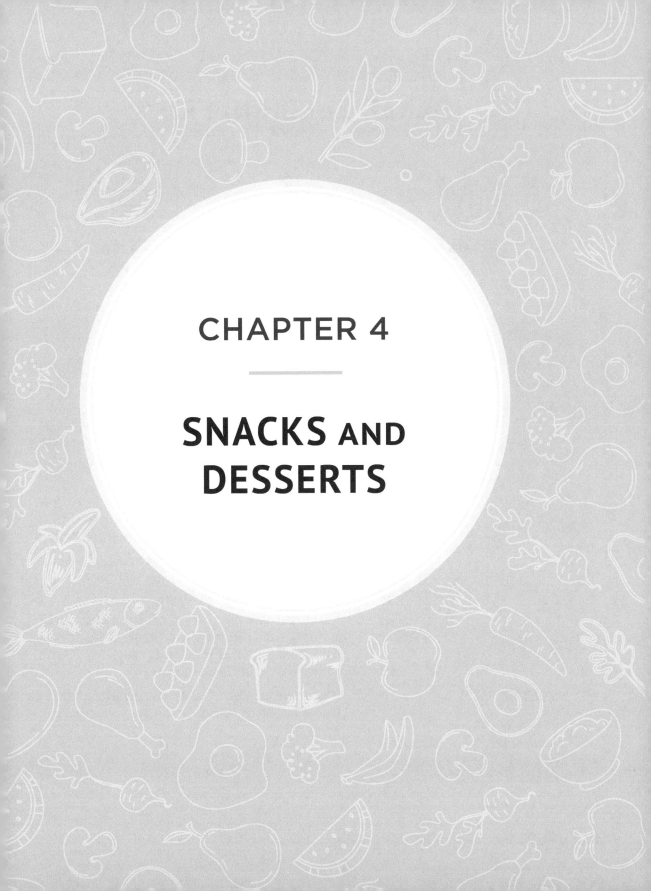

# CHAPTER 4

---

## SNACKS AND DESSERTS

# BAKED ZUCCHINI FRIES

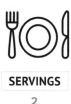

**SERVINGS**
2

**PREP TIME**
10 MIN

**COOK TIME**
23 MIN

## INGREDIENTS

- 2 medium zucchinis
- ½ cup dairy-free parmesan cheese or ¼ cup nutritional yeast
- 1 large egg
- ¼ teaspoon asafoetida (optional)
- ½ teaspoon salt

## DIRECTIONS

1. Preheat the oven to 425 degrees F. and line a baking sheet with parchment paper. Set aside.

2. Cut each zucchini in half lengthwise and then half again (to make eight long sticks). Then cut the sticks once crosswise, making 16 sticks from each squash.

3. In a medium bowl, combine the dairy-free parmesan cheese, salt, and asafoetida (optional). Whisk egg in a separate bowl.

4. Dip each zucchini stick in the egg, shake off the excess, then press into the parmesan mixture, coating all sides.

5. Place the zucchini fries on the prepared baking sheet in a single layer. Bake for 10 minutes. Flip the fries and bake for 10 more minutes, or until golden.

6. Place under the broiler for about 2 to 3 minutes, until darker golden and crispy. Enjoy!

### NUTRITION FACTS

**Per serving:** (8 sticks)
Calories: 123; Total fat: 5g; Protein: 11g; Carbohydrates: 5g; Fiber: 2.5g

# KALE CHIPS

**SERVINGS**

2

**PREP TIME**

5 MIN

**COOK TIME**

15 MIN

## INGREDIENTS

- 1 bunch kale, stemmed and coarsely chopped
- 1 tablespoon olive oil
- ½ teaspoon salt
- ¼ teaspoon ground cumin (optional)

## DIRECTIONS

1. Preheat the oven to 350 degrees F. and line a baking sheet with parchment paper. Set aside.
2. In a large bowl, toss the kale with the olive oil, salt, and cumin (optional). Spread the kale in a single layer on the prepared baking sheet.
3. Bake until the kale is crisp but not burnt, about 15 minutes.
4. Remove from the oven and let cool slightly (chips will crisp up even more once out of the oven). Enjoy!

**NUTRITION FACTS**

**Per serving:** (½ of recipe)
Calories: 63; Total fat: 6g; Protein: 0g; Carbohydrates: 0g; Fiber: 0g

# GLUTEN-FREE CRACKERS

**SERVINGS**

12

**PREP TIME**

20 MIN

**COOK TIME**

22 MIN

## INGREDIENTS

- ¾ cup gluten-free flour blend
- ⅔ cup blanched almond flour
- 2 tablespoons avocado oil or neutral coconut oil
- 2 tablespoons flaxseed meal
- 1 teaspoon fresh chopped rosemary
- ¼ teaspoon baking powder
- ¼ teaspoon asafetida (optional)
- ½ teaspoon salt

### NUTRITION FACTS

**Per serving:** (5 crackers)
Calories: 85; Total fat: 5.6g;
Protein: 1g; Carbohydrates:
6g; Fiber: 1g

## DIRECTIONS

1. Preheat the oven to 325 degrees F. and line a large baking sheet with parchment paper.

2. Add all ingredients (except the oil) to a food processor or a mixing bowl and process or whisk until thoroughly combine. Add oil and pulse or use a fork until crumbly or mixture is a coarse blend.

3. Add a tablespoon of water at a time and pulse or stir until a semi-sticky dough forms. Don't add more than 5 tablespoons of water.

4. Remove from food processor or mixing bowl and form into a loose ball. Press using a rolling pin between 2 pieces of parchment paper to ⅛-inch thickness.

5. Transfer the bottom piece of parchment paper with rolled out dough onto a baking sheet. Cut the dough into 1-inch squares with a pizza cutter or a knife.

6. Bake for about 16 to 22 minutes, until the crackers are light golden brown.

7. Remove from the oven and let cool for 10 minutes before gently separating them. Cool completely before serving.

# BAKED POTATO FRIES

**SERVINGS**
2

**PREP TIME**
10 MIN

**COOK TIME**
20 MIN

## INGREDIENTS

- 1 large potato, peeled and cut into ¼-inch sticks
- 1 tablespoon extra virgin olive oil
- ½ teaspoon salt

## DIRECTIONS

1. Preheat the oven to 425 degrees F. and line a baking sheet with parchment paper. Set aside.

2. Fill a medium bowl with cold water and let potatoes soak in water for at least 30 minutes (this helps to remove excess starch). Remove from water and dry very well using absorbent paper towels.

3. In a medium bowl, add the potato sticks and toss with olive oil and salt.

4. Spread evenly in a single layer on the prepared baking sheet. Make sure they are in a single layer and are not piled up.

5. Bake for about 15-20 minutes, turning after the first 10 minutes, until crispy and the edges are golden brown. Watch them carefully to avoid burning.

6. Remove from the oven and let cool a few minutes. Sprinkle with salt and enjoy!

## NUTRITION FACTS

**Per serving:** (½ of recipe)
Calories: 115; Total fat: 6.8g;
Protein: 1g; Carbohydrates:
11g; Fiber: 2g

# BROCCOLI TOTS

**SERVINGS**

2

**PREP TIME**

15 MIN

**COOK TIME**

25 MIN

## INGREDIENTS

- 3 cups fresh or frozen broccoli florets
- 1 large egg
- 1 egg white
- ⅓ cup grated dairy-free parmesan cheese (or any dairy-free cheese alternative can work)
- 4 tablespoons almond flour (or oat flour)
- 1 teaspoon dried oregano
- 1 teaspoon dried parsley
- ½ teaspoon asafoetida (optional)
- ½ teaspoon salt

**NUTRITION FACTS**

**Per serving:** (4 tots)
Calories: 102; Total fat: 5.7g;
Protein: 7g; Carbohydrates:
3.7g; Fiber: 2g

## DIRECTIONS

1. Preheat the oven to 400 degrees F. and line a baking sheet with parchment paper. Set aside.

2. Steam broccoli for about 3-5 minutes and then rinse with cold water to stop the cooking process. Drain well and dry broccoli with paper towel.

3. Finely chop the cooked broccoli using a knife. Alternatively, you can use a food processor and pulse the broccoli until it's finely chopped.

4. Add broccoli to a large bowl and mix with eggs, dairy-free parmesan cheese, almond flour, oregano, parsley, salt, and asafoetida (if using).

5. Using a heaping tablespoon, scoop about 1 ½ – 2 tablespoons of the mixture into the palm of your hand. Gently mold into a tater-tot shape ball. Place onto prepared baking sheet.

6. Bake for 10 minutes, turning them over and bake for a remaining 10-15 minutes until golden brown. Enjoy!

# BANANA BREAD MUFFINS

**SERVINGS**

10

**PREP TIME**

15 MIN

**COOK TIME**

25 MIN

## INGREDIENTS

- 3 medium ripe bananas, mashed (1 ½ cups approx.)
- 1 ¾ cups gluten-free all-purpose flour
- ¼ cup almond milk or other plant-based milk
- ¼ cup melted coconut oil
- ¼ maple syrup or honey (see note)
- 1 large egg, beaten
- 1 teaspoon baking soda
- ½ teaspoons baking powder
- 1 teaspoon vanilla extract (optional)
- ¼ teaspoon salt

### NUTRITION FACTS

**Per serving:** (1 muffin)
Calories: 152; Total fat: 5.4g;
Protein: 1g; Carbohydrates:
23g; Fiber: 1g

## DIRECTIONS

1. Preheat the oven to 350 degrees F. Spray a 12-count muffin pan with nonstick cooking spray or use cupcake liners.
2. Whisk together flour, baking soda, baking powder, and salt in a medium bowl. Set aside.
3. In a large bowl, combine the coconut oil and coconut sugar or maple syrup. Add the egg, mashed banana, almond milk, and vanilla (if using). Mix well.
4. Add dry ingredients and mix just until combined.
5. Pour the mixture into prepared muffin pan and bake for 20-25 minutes, or until a toothpick inserted into a muffin comes out clean.
6. Place the muffin tin on a cooling rack to cool.

### NOTE

If you use ripe-enough bananas, you may not have to add any sweetener to your muffins. You can also substitute maple syrup and honey for monk fruit or even stevia.

# COCONUT COOKIES

**SERVINGS**
18

**PREP TIME**
20 MIN

**COOK TIME**
12 MIN

## INGREDIENTS

- 1 ripe banana, mashed
- 1 cup gluten-free all-purpose flour
- ½ cup unsweetened coconut flakes
- ½ cup oat flour
- 1 large egg
- 1 egg white
- 2 tablespoons melted coconut oil
- ¼ cup maple syrup
- ½ cup pitted dates, chopped
- ½ teaspoon baking powder
- 1 teaspoon vanilla extract
- ¼ teaspoon salt

### NUTRITION FACTS

**Per serving:** (1 large cookie) Calories: 92; Total fat: 2.7g; Protein: 1.5g; Carbohydrates: 14g; Fiber: 1.5g

## DIRECTIONS

1. Preheat the oven to 350°F. Line a large baking sheet with parchment paper. Set aside.

2. In a medium bowl, combine together the mashed banana, coconut oil, maple syrup, eggs, and vanilla.

3. In a separate bowl, sift together the gluten-free flour, oat flour, salt, and baking powder.

4. Mix the wet and dry ingredients until combined then stir in the dates and coconut flakes. Cover and place in the refrigerator for 30 minutes.

5. Roll or scoop the dough into 2 tablespoons portions and place them a couple inches apart on the prepared baking sheets. Press the top of each ball of dough to flatten slightly.

6. Bake for about 9 to 12 minutes, until the edges are just beginning to turn golden brown. Remove from the oven and transfer the cookies to wire racks to cool completely.

# CAROB BROWNIES

**SERVINGS**

9

**PREP TIME**

15 MIN

**COOK TIME**

30 MIN

## INGREDIENTS

- ¾ cup gluten-free all-purpose flour
- 5 tablespoons carob powder
- 1 large egg
- 1 egg white
- ½ cups maple syrup or honey
- 2 tablespoons coconut oil
- 2 tablespoons unsweetened applesauce
- ½ teaspoon baking soda
- 1 teaspoon vanilla extract
- ¼ teaspoon salt

## DIRECTIONS

1. Preheat the oven to 325 degrees F. Grease an 8x8-inch baking pan. Set aside.

2. In a medium bowl, mix together the flour, carob powder, baking soda, and salt. In a separate bowl, mix wet ingredients.

3. Add dry ingredients to wet ingredients and mix until combined.

4. Pour the mixture into the prepared baking pan and bake for 25 to 30 minutes, or until toothpick comes out clean when inserted into middle of brownies.

5. Let cool and cut into squares.

### NUTRITION FACTS

**Per serving:** (1 slice)
Calories: 128; Total fat: 3.7g; Protein: 1.7g; Carbohydrates: 21g; Fiber: 1g

# WATERMELON SORBET

**SERVINGS**

1

**PREP TIME**

10 MIN

**COOK TIME**

N/A

## INGREDIENTS

- 2 cups fresh seedless watermelon chunks
- ⅔ cup unsweetened coconut milk
- 2 teaspoons maple syrup or honey
- 1-inch ginger, peeled and grated

## DIRECTIONS

1. Dice the fresh watermelon into 1-2-inch cubes. Measure out about 2 cups and place the pieces in the freezer overnight.

2. In a blender, add the watermelon, coconut milk, ginger, and maple syrup. Pulse 10 times, until combined, then stop the blender and stir mixture with a spoon.

3. Blend ingredients on high power until smooth, adding more coconut milk if needed.

4. Serve immediately for a softer texture, or transfer into a freezer-safe container and freeze for about 3-4 hours or until firm.

**NUTRITION FACTS**

**Per serving:** (2 cups)
Calories: 139; Total fat: 3.3g;
Protein: 1.5g; Carbohydrates:
27g; Fiber: 1g

# SPIRULINA NICE CREAM

**SERVINGS**

2

**PREP TIME**

10 MIN

**COOK TIME**

N/A

## INGREDIENTS

- 3 ripe bananas, sliced and frozen
- ¼ cup almond milk or other plant-based milk
- 1 teaspoon blue or green spirulina

## DIRECTIONS

1. Remove the sliced frozen bananas from the freezer and let them thaw for 5 minutes.

2. In a blender, combine the bananas, almond milk, and spirulina, and blend on high speed until soft and creamy. Use a tamper to push down ingredients into blender while on. This helps to ensure the bananas and other ingredients are adequately pulverized.

3. Serve immediately or store in a freezer safe container until ready to enjoy.

**NUTRITION FACTS**

**Per serving:** (1 cup approx.)
Calories: 168; Total fat: 1g;
Protein: 2.6g; Carbohydrates:
37g; Fiber: 4.7g

# CHAPTER 5

---

# SMOOTHIES AND BEVERAGES

# BANANA MANGO SMOOTHIE

**SERVINGS**

1

**PREP TIME**

5 MIN

**COOK TIME**

N/A

## INGREDIENTS

- 1 medium banana, sliced
- ¼ cup fresh or frozen mango
- ½ teaspoon fresh ginger, grated
- ½ cup almond milk or other plant-based milk

## DIRECTIONS

1. Add all ingredients to a blender and process until smooth, adding more almond milk if needed to get your desired texture.

2. Serve immediately and enjoy!

**NUTRITION FACTS**

**Per serving:** (1 cup)
Calories: 158; Total fat: 1.8g;
Protein: 2.2g; Carbohydrates:
33g; Fiber: 4g

# STRAWBERRY BEET SMOOTHIE

**SERVINGS**

2

**PREP TIME**

5 MIN

**COOK TIME**

N/A

## INGREDIENTS

- 1 cup beets, chopped (preferably cooked)
- 1 cup almond milk
- ½ cup frozen strawberries
- 1 tablespoon maple syrup or honey

## DIRECTIONS

1. Combine all the ingredients in a blender and blend until smooth.
2. Pour into glasses and enjoy.

**NUTRITION FACTS**

**Per serving:** (1 cup)
Calories: 89; Total fat: 1g;
Protein: 2g; Carbohydrates:
17g; Fiber: 2.6g

# WATERMELON CUCUMBER JUICE

**SERVINGS**

1

**PREP TIME**

5 MIN

**COOK TIME**

N/A

## INGREDIENTS

- 1 ½ cups watermelon, seedless and cubed
- ½ cup English cucumber, sliced
- 1 teaspoon chia seeds
- ½ teaspoon lemon zest (optional)

## DIRECTIONS

1. Add the watermelon, cucumber, and lemon zest to a blender, and blend until smooth.
2. Strain the juice through a fine mesh sieve or cheese cloth to remove the pulp.
3. Stir in chia and chill the juice for at least 20 minutes. Enjoy!

**NUTRITION FACTS**

**Per serving:** (2 cups)
Calories: 76; Total fat: 1g;
Protein: 3g; Carbohydrates:
12g; Fiber: 3g

# MELON SMOOTHIE

**SERVINGS**

2

**PREP TIME**

5 MIN

**COOK TIME**

N/A

## INGREDIENTS

- 1 ½ cups cantaloupe, chopped (you can use other melon too)
- 1 ½ cups almond milk or other plant-based milk
- ½ cup plain non-dairy yogurt (optional)
- 1 tablespoon maple syrup

## DIRECTIONS

1. Combine all the ingredients in a blender and blend until smooth.
2. Pour into glasses and enjoy.

### NUTRITION FACTS

**Per serving:** (1 ¾ cups)
Calories: 155; Total fat: 3.6g;
Protein: 2g; Carbohydrates:
29g; Fiber: 2g

# CAROB BANANA SMOOTHIE

**SERVINGS**

1

**PREP TIME**

5 MIN

**COOK TIME**

N/A

## INGREDIENTS

- 1 frozen banana
- ½ cup almond milk or other plant-based milk
- 1 tablespoon carob powder
- 1 tablespoon almond butter
- 1 tablespoon maple syrup or honey (optional)

## DIRECTIONS

1. Place all ingredients into a blender and blend until smooth. If you prefer a thinner smoothie, add more milk to get the desired texture.

2. Serve immediately and enjoy!

**NUTRITION FACTS**

**Per serving:** (1 ¾ cups)
Calories: 155; Total fat: 3.6g; Protein: 2g; Carbohydrates: 29g; Fiber: 2g

# CHAMOMILE LATTE

**SERVINGS**
2

**PREP TIME**
5 MIN

**COOK TIME**
10 MIN

## INGREDIENTS

- 1 ½ cups water
- 1 ½ cup almond milk or other plant-based milk
- 2 chamomile tea bags (or 2 teaspoons loose leaf tea)
- 4 cloves, crushed (see note)
- 1 cinnamon stick (see note)
- 1 tablespoon maple syrup or honey

## DIRECTIONS

1. Bring the water to a simmer in a small saucepan. Once boiling, add chamomile, cinnamon stick, and cloves. Remove from heat and cover, letting steep for 10 minutes.

2. Meanwhile, heat the milk in another small saucepan over medium heat. Whisk constantly until warn and frothy, about 5 minutes.

3. Discard the tea bags, cinnamon stick, and cloves from the saucepan of tea (you can use a mesh strainer). Stir in honey and top with the warm, frothy milk.

4. Serve immediately.

**NUTRITION FACTS**

**Per serving:** (1 ½ cups approx.) Calories: 67; Total fat: 1.9g; Protein: 0g; Carbohydrates: 12g; Fiber: 0g

**NOTE**

Heating spices such as cinnamon and cloves effectively dampens their carminative effect while maintaining its distinctive flavor. However, if you have a problem with these spices, you can leave them out.

# APPLE CARROT BEET JUICE

**SERVINGS**

1

**PREP TIME**

10 MIN

**COOK TIME**

N/A

## INGREDIENTS

- 1 Red Delicious apple, peeled, cored and quartered
- 1 small beet, cut into chunks (see note)
- 1-2 medium carrots, peeled and ends trimmed
- ½ teaspoon fresh ginger, peeled
- ½ cup water

## DIRECTIONS

1. Place all ingredients in a blender and blend until smooth, about 1-2 minutes. Use the tamper if needed.

2. Place a fine mesh strainer over a large bowl and pour the juice over. Press the pulp down and squeeze all of the juice out.

3. Discard the pulp and pour the juice into a serving glass. Drink immediately or chill in the fridge to enjoy later.

### NUTRITION FACTS

**Per serving:** (1 cup approx.)
Calories: 210; Total fat: 1g;
Protein: 3g; Carbohydrates:
38g; Fiber: 2g

### NOTE

If you can't tolerate raw beet juice, you can steam the beet before adding it to the blender with the other ingredients.

# PEAR GINGER SMOOTHIE

**SERVINGS**

2

**PREP TIME**

10 MIN

**COOK TIME**

N/A

## INGREDIENTS

- 2 ripe Bosc pears, peeled and cut into chunks
- 1 cup almond milk or other plant-based milk
- ½ cup plain non-dairy yogurt
- 1-2 teaspoons fresh ginger, grated

## DIRECTIONS

1. Place all ingredients into a blender and blend until smooth.
2. Serve immediately and enjoy!

**NUTRITION FACTS**

**Per serving:** (1 cup)
Calories: 189; Total fat: 3g; Protein: 1g; Carbohydrates: 32g; Fiber: 6.6g

**NOTE**

If you'd like a sweeter smoothie, you can add 1 tablespoon of maple syrup or honey.

# CHICORY LATTE

**SERVINGS**
1

**PREP TIME**
10 MIN

**COOK TIME**
5 MIN

## INGREDIENTS

- 1 teaspoon chicory root powder
- 1 cup water
- ¼ cup coconut milk or other plant-based milk
- 1 teaspoon coconut oil
- 1 teaspoon unflavored gelatin
- 1 teaspoon maple syrup or honey
- ½ teaspoon carob powder (optional)

## DIRECTIONS

1. Pour water into a coffee maker and brew the chicory brew. Alternatively, you can add the chicory to boiling water in a small pot or tea kettle and let steep for 7-10 minutes and then strain.

2. Once chicory root is steeped, add to a blender (you can use a hand blender too) along with coconut milk, coconut oil, maple syrup, gelatin and carob (if using) and blend on high-speed for a minute, until frothy.

3. Serve warm and enjoy!

**NUTRITION FACTS**

**Per serving:** (1 cup)
Calories: 134; Total fat: 5.6g;
Protein: 4.3g; Carbohydrates:
16g; Fiber: 1g

# PAPAYA ALOE VERA SMOOTHIE

**SERVINGS**

1

**PREP TIME**

5 MIN

**COOK TIME**

N/A

## INGREDIENTS

- 1 cup frozen papaya, cubed
- 1 cup unsweetened almond milk
- 2-4 ounces aloe vera gel (optional, but recommended)
- 1 tablespoon maple syrup or honey

## DIRECTIONS

1. Place all ingredients into a blender and blend until smooth.
2. Pour into a large glass and enjoy!

**NUTRITION FACTS**

**Per serving:** (2 cups)
Calories: 203; Total fat: 3g;
Protein: 2g; Carbohydrates:
40g; Fiber: 5g

# MEASUREMENTS AND CONVERSIONS

## VOLUMEN EQUIVALENTS (LIQUID)

| US STANDARDS | US STANDARDS (OUNCES) | METRIC (APPROX.) |
| --- | --- | --- |
| 2 tablespoons | 1 fl. oz. | 30 mL |
| ¼ cup | 2 fl. oz. | 60 mL |
| ½ cup | 4 fl. oz. | 120 mL |
| 1 cup | 8 fl. oz. | 240 mL |
| 1 ½ cups | 12 fl. oz. | 355 mL |
| 2 cups or 1 pint | 16 fl. oz. | 475 mL |
| 4 cups or 1 quart | 32 fl. oz. | 1 L |
| 1 gallon | 128 fl. oz. | 4 L |

## VOLUMEN EQUIVALENTS (DRY)

| US STANDARDS | METRIC (APPROX.) |
| --- | --- |
| ⅛ teaspoon | 0.5 mL |
| ¼ teaspoon | 1 mL |
| ½ teaspoon | 2 mL |
| ¾ teaspoon | 4 mL |
| 1 teaspoon | 5 mL |
| 1 tablespoon | 15 mL |
| ¼ cup | 59 mL |
| ⅓ cup | 79 mL |

| | |
|---|---|
| ½ cup | 118 mL |
| ⅔ cup | 156 mL |
| ¾ cup | 177 mL |
| 1 cup | 235 mL |
| 2 cups or 1 pint | 475 mL |
| 3 cups | 700 mL |
| 4 cups or 1 quart | 1 L |

## WEIGHT EQUIVALENTS

| US STANDARD | METRIC (APPROX.) |
|---|---|
| ½ ounce | 15 g |
| 1 ounce | 30 g |
| 2 ounces | 60 g |
| 4 ounces | 115 g |
| 8 ounces | 190°C |
| 12 ounces | 225 g |
| 16 ounces or 1 pound | 340 g |

## OVEN TEMPERATURES

| FAHRENHEIT (F) | CELSIUS (C) (APPROX.) |
|---|---|
| 250°F | 120°C |
| 300°F | 150°C |
| 325°F | 165°C |
| 350°F | 180°C |
| 375°F | 190°C |
| 400°F | 200°C |
| 425°F | 220°C |
| 450°F | 230°C |

# ABOUT THE AUTHOR

**L. G. Capellan** is a voracious researcher of digestive problems, with extensive experience and knowledge about gastritis and bile reflux. In 2013, he was diagnosed with chronic gastritis, acid reflux, and bile reflux—digestive problems that he suffered from for several years until he decided to take his health in his own hands and do things on his own.

He spent more than 5 years researching a solution to his chronic gastritis and bile reflux. This included dedicating thousands of hours to reading medical and scientific research, articles on blogs and websites, and gastritis success stories on online health forums. His deep research provided him with a new understanding of what he had to do, how, and in what order to heal his gastritis and digestive problems.

Now, through his Facebook group (*The Gastritis Healing Group*) and his book about gastritis, he helps other people who are going through the same situation he once went through, so that they can also get rid of gastritis and take back their health.

To contact or connect with the author, go to next page to find contact details.

# CONTACT AND FOLLOW

The best way to contact the author is via email at contact@lgcapellan.com and you can also:

## Join his Community on Facebook:

www.facebook.com/groups/thegastritishealingroup

## Follow him on Social Media:

Facebook - www.facebook.com/lgcapellan.author
Twitter - www.twitter.com/lg_capellan
Instagram - www.instagram.com/lg_capellan

## Find More Info on his Website:

www.lgcapellan.com

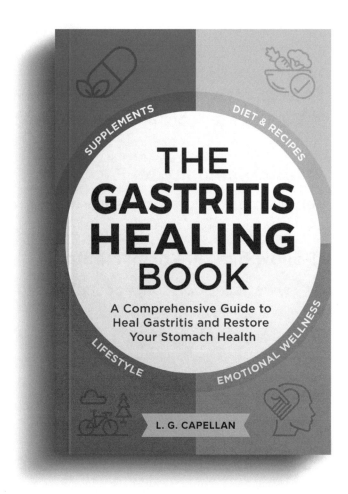

Manufactured by Amazon.ca
Bolton, ON

29291609R00042